Developing Care Pathways

The Tool Kit

Kathryn de Lúc

In collaboration with

Denise Kitchiner
Amanda Layton
Elaine Morris
Yvonne Murray
and
Sue Overill

National Pathways Association

Radcliffe Medical P

Radcliffe Medical Press Ltd
18 Marcham Road, Abingdon, Oxon OX14 1AA

British Library Cataloguing in Publication Data

A catalogue record for this book is available from the British Library.

ISBN 1 85775 499 9

Typeset by Joshua Associates Ltd, Oxford
Printed and bound by Hobbs the Printers, Totton, Hants

Contents

Chapter 1

Introduction

So you want to develop care pathways . . . but you don't know where to start.

The purpose of this Tool Kit is to provide you with the information you need to help you develop care pathways. It is meant to be a practical reference, which anyone undertaking the development of care pathways can use as a source of advice and expertise.

What is required?

1 A facilitator who has credibility.
2 Establishment of a multidisciplinary group of staff (these need to be staff who are actually involved in the 'hands-on' delivery of care support for the particular topic chosen, including junior medical staff, consultants, staff nurses, GP practice nurses, etc.) and non-clinical staff as required.
3 Resources to support the development process (e.g. production of new care pathway documentation, notes of development meetings, etc.).

A number of different steps have been identified in the development, implementation and maintenance process for individual care pathways. These are outlined in this Tool Kit. Additional information about care pathways is outlined in the Handbook of this resource guide.

Chapter 2

Development of your care pathway

Select a topic

It is advisable to involve the team who will be developing the care pathway in deciding the topic. Some suggested criteria to help choose a topic are listed below:

- simple condition (for an early success)
- clinical staff express a desire for development
- identify a problem(s) or reason for developing it
- the area chosen has clear start and end points
- subject of national guideline/policy initiative
- area at risk of service fragmentation.

In addition, some suggest you should choose conditions which are:

- common, high percentage of patients/users (greatest impact in organisation) and/or high cost
- high clinical variability in treatment and outcomes
- conditions requiring many interventions.

Box 2.1: Choosing a topic for your care pathway

Topic example:

- cataract operation
- hospital-at-home
- anxiety management.

Now you choose the topic for your care pathway.

Topic chosen:

The multidisciplinary development group

The establishment of a multidisciplinary group to develop the care pathway is recommended. Exclusion of any group of staff involved in the provision of care for the patient/user group covered by the care pathway is likely to result in ownership problems later. Staff who do not have direct involvement in the care pathway development are likely to question the content of the care pathway if it does not represent familiar practice.

Consider involving patient/user or consumer representative groups in your development meetings as well as commissioners and representatives from other agencies (e.g. social services). It may also be relevant to involve non-clinical staff such as porters, domestics, administrative and clerical staff if changes in services proposed involve these support services. Also, consider involving clinical audit staff, risk management and directorate managers to make sure the care pathway changes are integrated into other things.

Identify below the individual members of the multidisciplinary group that will develop your care pathway. It is advised that this group is not too large – say 10–15 members.

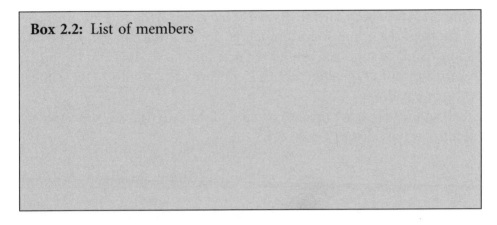

Box 2.2: List of members

Role of the representative on the multidisciplinary development group

As a representative on the multidisciplinary development group, an individual will perform essentially four roles. These are:

- provide detailed knowledge of what happens locally now
- provide an 'expert knowledge' base about the particular selected topic
- challenge clinical colleagues
- discuss with peers who are not present at the development meetings the proposed content of the care pathway. Some organisations have found the formation of 'consensus' groups useful to ensure wider debate and agreement to particular aspects of a care pathway.

This last role is vital and is one that staff in the development groups do not always appreciate fully. Whilst many clinical staff are used to providing 'expert knowledge/experience' within a group, not all of them may appreciate the importance of feeding back and checking out with their colleagues what the group is doing. This role is important, as it helps the other clinical staff develop ownership of the care pathway as it is developed.

Recording the decisions taken by the development group

It is advisable to make a record of the discussions and major decisions taken as part of the development of the care pathway. This provides a useful reference, both for the development group itself and for others, to see the steps the group went through in deciding the content of the care pathway and the rationale behind the decisions taken. It is also important to keep a record of the literature and evidence used to inform the content of the care pathway.

An outline template to record content of the care pathway development meetings is provided in Figure 2.1.

Box 2.3: Useful tips

- Keep meetings short (1 hour maximum).
- Keep meetings regular and frequent.
- Obtain commitment from those in the development group to develop the care pathway, i.e. get them to 'sign up' to the development.
- If the group gets too large, break it down into subgroups, but make sure the subgroups report regularly back to the main group.
- Continue to review the membership of the development group throughout the process of development. It is not unusual to find you have missed some staff groups out.

Identification of the scope of the care pathway

- Where will the care pathway begin and end?
- Which patients/users will it include or exclude?

Answering these questions will require discussion among the multi-disciplinary development group. The answers are likely to be influenced by what you are trying to achieve in developing the care pathway. For example, the desire to improve communication between primary care and hospital is likely to result in a care pathway crossing this traditional organisational boundary.

Date........   Meeting number ....   Stage in process ....

Present:

Discussion topic	Action/Decision agreed	Who to action
1		
2		
3		

Reference clinical evidence used:
(i) ....
(ii) ....
(iii) ....

Items for next meeting:

Items for future consideration:

Next meeting:
Date.......   Time ......   Location ....

Figure 2.1: Care pathway development meeting template.

You will need to identify inclusion or exclusion criteria for your care pathway at this point. It is important to include these criteria on any care pathway documentation developed subsequently, so that clinical staff are clear about the specific circumstances in which the individual care pathway should be applied.

An important consideration at this stage is to decide the type of grouping of patients/users for whom you wish to develop the care pathway. It could be:

- condition/disease-based – for example, diabetes, stroke
- symptom-based – for example, chest pain, panic attacks
- treatment/procedure/service-based – for example, hernia operation, hospital-at-home
- problem-based – for example, managing at home, smoking cessation
- some combination of these groupings (see below).

The facilitator needs to be vigilant in making sure that the clinical team tests the appropriateness of classification of patients/users to go on the care pathway. It is important to make sure patients/users will not be put on an inappropriate care pathway. For example, patients displaying symptoms but with no confirmed diagnosis should not be put onto a diagnosis-based pathway. Breaking down the care pathway into sections which can be slotted together to form building blocks which, when put together, will reflect the entire patient's/user's journey is one way of tackling this complexity. For example:

- *Stage one – symptom*: chest pain. Patients present with chest pain as a symptom. This will include patients who have had a myocardial infarction as well as patients who have other cardiac conditions.
- *Stage two – diagnosis*: myocardial infarction. Patients are confirmed as having had a myocardial infarction.
- *Stage three – programme*: cardiac rehabilitation. This will include patients who have had myocardial infarction as well as (possibly) other cardiac patients requiring rehabilitation.

Now you define the scope of the care pathway you want to develop in Box 2.4.

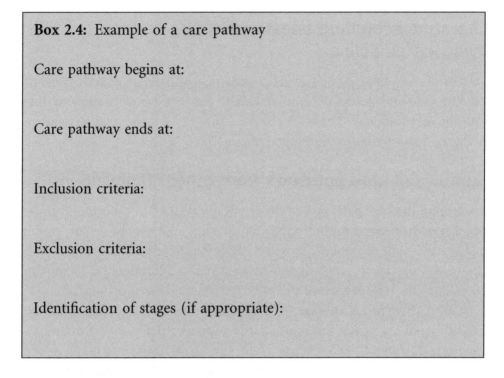

Obtaining information

Experience has shown that it is helpful to collect four types of information.
These are:

1 audit of current local practices (baseline review)
2 literature search on latest research, evidence/guidelines
3 samples of care pathways from other organisations
4 patient/user views on current services.

Audit of current local practices (baseline review)

An audit of the clinical records prior to the care pathway development will
provide information as to what happens now. It will also highlight any
problems or issues you want to tackle as part of the care pathway
development. This might include areas for streamlining, and removing
duplications or blocks in the process of care. It will also provide
information on whether outcome information is collected.

Literature search on latest research, evidence/guidelines

One of the key benefits of the development process is an examination of existing evidence/guidelines and research, and the incorporation of this into the care pathway. The evidence used should be referenced in the care pathway documentation developed later.

Samples of care pathways from other organisations

Examining the care pathways of other organisations has been found to be of great benefit to the multidisciplinary development group. It reduces the need to 'reinvent the wheel', provides ideas about content and format, and shows how particular issues like co-morbidities or additional problems can be dealt with. However, care pathway documentation is a by-product of reviewing the *process* of care. The facilitator needs to ensure that the multidisciplinary group does not simply copy another organisation's care pathway document. A key benefit of the development process is the detailed discussion that goes on between staff and the examination and review of local current practice. This discussion is vital to ensuring ownership of the changes in the *process* identified by the group developing the care pathway.

Patient/user information

Various mechanisms can be used to collect patient/user views on current services and their suggestions for improvements. These include:

- patient/user representation on the care pathway development group
- consumer group (e.g. community health council, Stroke Association, local support groups) representation on the care pathway development group
- patient/user focus group discussion/user forums
- telephone/postal surveys
- information from complaints.

See the section on the patient/user in the Handbook for more information on this.

Box 2.5: Useful tips

- Leave developing care pathways in areas of multiple pathology and complex conditions until you have gained experience in their development.
- If the pathway is long and complex, break down the pathway into sections and do a section at a time.
- Get the clinical staff to undertake the literature search for the evidence – this assists with the 'ownership'.
- If you have patient/user representation of the development group ensure you have more than one user. These groups can be intimidating to individuals not used to this environment.
- Visit other organisations to see how their care pathway works in practice.

Care pathway objectives

The multidisciplinary discussion will begin to identify the issues the group wants to tackle in the development of their care pathway. These issues should be translated into care pathway objectives and/or outcomes. Sometimes, issues are identified which have a much wider impact than on one single care pathway. For example, the need for a trust or GP practice-wide protocol might be identified. The development group needs to decide whether it should do this additional work or whether another group is better placed to carry out this additional task.

The care pathway objectives need to be specific. For example: 'improve the quality of healthcare' does not inform the content of the care pathway. Instead, you could have: *'improve the quality of healthcare by clarifying the information required by the district nurse team following the discharge of . . . patients/users from hospital'*. It might also help to get the staff to identify what are the problems with caring/treating for that particular set of patients/users that frustrate them now. Can these be translated into objectives for the care pathway to sort out?

The traditional principles about objective writing apply. The objectives need to be specific and measurable. The development group needs to identify how they will be measured and include a target for achievement.

Table 2.1: Example of objective setting – hernia day case care pathway

Objective	Measurement	Target
Reduce number of visits by patients to acute unit	Number of visits to acute unit	1
Elimination of unexpected overnight stays in acute unit	Number of overnight stays with reason	Nil
Improvement in patient's physical health following operation	Level of discomfort experienced by the patient caused by the hernia (questionnaire)	Improved score
Improvement or maintenance of patient's social health status following operation	Ability to undertake pastimes/hobbies Ability to return to work/ domestic chores (questionnaire e.g. SF36)	Improved score

Source: Worcestershire NHS Trust

Now you identify the objectives for your care pathway.

Objective/Outcome	Measurement	Target

Process mapping the care pathway

This is a vital part of the development of the care pathway and one that is often overlooked. It involves tracing the patient's/user's expected journey through the care process and requires the development of a process map. This is very similar to the drawing of a flow chart.

The process mapping allows the development group to see the 'whole picture' of the care process with all the major steps identified. It highlights the order in which things are completed or when specialists have their input. It also allows you to identify the standards of care you may wish to monitor at the various stages of care.

Ask the following questions:

- What are the interventions?
- When should the interventions be completed?
- Who should complete them?
- Where should they be completed?

It is possible to use the standard flow chart symbols to describe the care process for which you are writing your care pathway. For example, you can use the symbols:

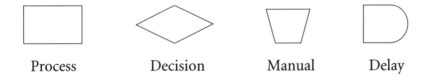

Process   Decision   Manual   Delay

When you have completed a process map for what happens now, draw another one detailing the changes you wish to make as part of the care pathway.

Much has been written about the technique of drawing flow charts in the quality literature. For more information on this subject a useful reference is:

- NHS Executive (1995) *Leading Improvement in Healthcare: a resource guide for process improvement.* DoH, London.

Box 2.6: Useful tips

- To help explain the concept of 'process mapping' to staff try drawing a process map of a routine domestic chore, for example 'getting up in the morning and going to work.' Identify the key steps, e.g. getting dressed, eating breakfast, etc. Outline the consequences if some key steps are not followed in a logical order.

- Consider inserting the 'process map' at the beginning of the care pathway documentation. This helps staff see the overview of the care pathway when using the documentation.

Draw the 'process map' of what happens now for the patients/users for whom you wish to develop the care pathway. Identify the changes you want to make to the process to improve the care delivered as part of the care pathway. This will involve redrawing the process map to reflect the planned changes.

Programme of development for an individual care pathway

As with any change management project involving changes in practice, there needs to be discussion and a consensus reached regarding the content of the individual care pathway. This makes it very difficult to estimate the time and number of meetings it will take to develop a single care pathway. A suggested programme of development meetings is set out on p. 16. Use this programme as a guide to decide the order in which topics should be discussed within the multidisciplinary development group.

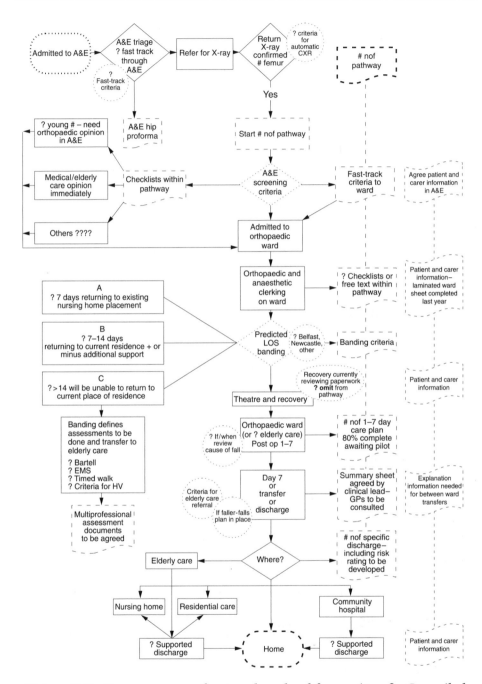

Figure 2.2: Process map – fractured neck of femur (#nof). Compiled for educational and consultation purposes by the Directorate for Clinical Effectiveness, Salisbury Health Care NHS Trust, June 2000. *Source:* Salisbury Health Care NHS Trust.

First meeting

- Get members of development group to 'sign up' to the principle of development.
- Confirm role of development group and individual members.
- Confirm topic and scope of care pathway.
- Check membership of development group reflects all disciplines/agencies involved.
- Identify current problems/issues in topic area.
- Agree information to be available for the next meeting, including latest evidence and guidelines, audit results of current service, patient/user views, other sample care pathways.

Second meeting

- Identify objectives for care pathway.
- Identify outcomes to be measured as part of care pathway.
- Draw detailed 'process map' of current service.
- Identify changes in service to be made.

Third meeting

- Agree revised 'process map' with planned changes in service, objectives and outcomes identified.
- Agree accompaniments to care pathway, e.g. new protocols/policies, patient/user booklets, measurement tools to be inserted into care pathway (satisfaction questionnaire, clinical tools, patient/user outcome tools etc.).
- Identify training requirements resulting from planned changes in service.

Fourth meeting

- Agree principles for care pathway documentation (where kept, documentation template and style, system for recording variations, how to integrate different disciplines notes, practicalities of producing documentation, etc.).
- Agree who will draft out documentation.

Fifth meeting

- Agree draft care pathway documentation (this may take several redrafts).
- Set date and timescale for pilot of care pathway.
- Agree support arrangements for staff during pilot.
- Agree training plan for staff to use the care pathway.
- Agree how variations will be audited.
- Agree feedback date for results of pilot.

Check list for the development of an individual care pathway

Table 2.2 is a check list of all the information required relating to the care pathway development.

Table 2.2: Check list for care pathway development

Feature to check	Checked
• Has the membership of the development group been identified?	☐
• Have you identified a care pathway topic?	☐
• Have you identified objectives/outcomes for your care pathway?	☐
• Have you identified inclusion criteria?	☐
• Have you identified exclusion criteria?	☐
• Have you identified the start point of your care pathway?	☐
• Have you identified the end point of your care pathway?	☐
• Within which geographical areas/location will the care pathway be implemented?	☐
• Is there a lead person identified for the care pathway?	☐
• Have patient/user views been incorporated into the care pathway?	☐
• Has a process map been drawn for your care pathway?	☐
• Has a baseline audit of the care provided been undertaken?	☐
• Have sample pathways been reviewed from other organisations?	☐
• Has a literature search of the relevant evidence been completed?	☐
• Has a review of patient/user information been completed?	☐
• Which relevant guidelines, policies, procedures are referenced in the care pathway?	☐
• Have you incorporated assessment tools, charts and questionnaires into your care pathway?	☐

Source: Adapted from Worcestershire Acute Hospitals NHS Trust.

Chapter 3

Care pathway documentation

You might find it useful to read Chapter 2, *The legal aspects of care pathways* in the Handbook in conjunction with this section.

Computerised care pathways

The NPA believes that electronic care pathways (e-CPs) can be developed, which will have many advantages over the traditional paper-based care pathway documentation. However, to date there are very few examples in the UK where this type of development has occurred. Consequently, this part of the Tool Kit is written from the perspective of paper-based care pathways, although it is believed many of the principles are transferable to computerised care pathways.

Implications for staff

The design of the documentation is a *critical success factor*, which will have an impact on whether a care pathway is successfully introduced into an organisation. The fact is that the care pathway documentation:

- forms the *actual clinical record*
- is *multidisciplinary*
- *replaces existing clinical documentation*, e.g. nursing care plans, medical notes

These are three changes which often cause staff anxiety when designing the documentation.

Staff will have to change:

- the style with which they document care
- adopt a highly structured documentation format (template/prompts)
- abandon their own disciplines' specific documentation
- move to a multidisciplinary design.

These changes are likely to involve changes in where the documentation is kept.

Baseline audit

It is useful to undertake a baseline review of current documentation. This will identify any deficiencies that may exist in the documentation used pre-care pathway development.

Table 3.1: Baseline audit

Items to check	Checked
• Identify what information items are missing	☐
• Identify any unnecessary duplications of information	☐
• Is the plan of care kept up to date; is it timely and multidisciplinary?	☐
• Does the documentation reflect what actually happens – could it stand up in a court of law?	☐
• How many pages are used?	☐
• Do different people record the same information?	☐
• Can the documentation be used as an education tool for students?	☐
• Who writes in which parts of the notes?	☐
• Are all the notes stored together? If not, in how many locations are different sections stored?	☐
• Can variations from normal practice be identified?	☐

What to record

The aim is for the care pathway to guide clinical staff in 'what to do' not 'how to do it'. Care pathways therefore can and should reference other local policies/guidelines in use in the organisation. In this way, the care pathway remains concise.

Try to avoid the care pathway documentation becoming simply a list of tasks. Try to make it more outcomes-focused. For example, instead of having as a prompt 'check wound' have 'wound is dry'.

Many care pathway sites keep a limited space for free-text note taking. However, care must be taken to avoid this becoming the main part of the documentation and of staff repeating information in the free-text section which is in a prompt or more structured part of the documentation.

Guidelines for inclusion in the documentation

A few simple guidelines on care pathway documentation are listed below. The documentation should:

- form all or part of the clinical documentation
- replace existing documentation and *not* duplicate it
- be kept short and concise
- include information on date developed, date to be reviewed, version number and reference the guidelines/evidence used
- identify a space for the people completing the documentation to state their name, designation and signature
- have patient/user identifier information on every page
- assign accountability for completion of documentation
- ensure variation information can be easily captured and utilised
- be user-friendly.

Standardised format of documentation

An examination of the care pathways of different organisations shows that often, each individual care pathway has its own layout and style of documentation. This variability reflects the need to develop the 'owner-ship' by the group of staff who are both developing the care pathway and will be using it as their principal record of care. However, a balance should be struck between this variability and a standardised format.

Has your programme steering group developed a template of care pathway documentation, which will form a standard for all care pathways, developed within your organisation(s)? If not, consider asking it to do so. Staff will find a standardised format less confusing when multiple care pathways are being used.

Where to keep the documentation

The decision on where to keep the documentation depends on what is practical and workable in the local circumstances in order to maintain appropriate confidentiality and what the patient/user desires. As a principle, the NPA believes the documentation should be kept as close to the patient/user as possible.

Examples of where care pathways are kept include:

- with the patient/user
- at the foot or head of the bed
- in the clinical record folder.

It is also important to consider where the care pathway documentation will be kept once the pathway is completed. This is particularly relevant if the care pathway documentation crosses organisational boundaries.

Production of the documentation

Individuals frequently ask: 'Should the care pathway be printed or photocopied?'

There are advantages and disadvantages to both options but we would recommend that you do *not* consider printing your care pathway at least until it has been well tried and tested. It is very common for there to be a major review of the documentation (and particularly a slimming down of the content) 1–2 years after its introduction. Also, if the care pathway is being used to its full potential and the variations are being monitored and fed back to staff, then the content of the care pathway is likely to change. However, a photocopied document rarely looks as professional as one that has been printed and can result in the text being difficult to read, etc.

Some care pathway sites have found it useful to enlist the help of graphic designers to advise on the layout/font/use of colour, etc., in the documentation.

Box 3.1: Useful tips

- Leave the development of the documentation until completion of the 'process map' and the agreement of the changes in services which are going to result from the implementation of the care pathway.

- Make sure the care pathway documentation compliments any separate local initiative to improve clinical documentation, e.g. unified notes project.

- Collect all the separate pieces of paper used for documentation purposes pre-care pathway to compare with the amount of documentation included within the care pathway.

- Make sure you incorporate any 'house' or corporate style for the design of the documentation and the method for recording variations.

- The temptation at this stage (particularly if doing this for the first time) is to make the documentation record *everything*. It is easy to fall into the trap of recording explicitly what is implicit.

Chapter 4

Variation (or variance) reporting and analysis

What is variation reporting?

The concept of variation (exception) reporting (also known as variance reporting) is one of the most difficult aspects of care pathways to introduce successfully. Yet it probably offers the greatest potential benefits to both the staff using the care pathway and to the organisation. The term 'variation reporting' in the care pathway context should not be confused with the *statistical* process of variance analysis. Whilst you can produce statistical information from the analysis of the variations, this is only one product of recording the variations on the care pathway documentation.

Put simply, variation reporting is the difference between how patient/user care and outcomes are defined on the care pathway and what actually happens. The variation-reporting system allows staff to individualise the care pathway and take account of the individual requirements of each patient/user. If the care that is delivered varies from that outlined on the care pathway, this information **must** be recorded as a variation.

The variation-reporting element of a care pathway highlights the dynamic nature of the tool. The fact that variations will continue to be monitored and acted upon means a care pathway is never finalised. Continued refinement of the care pathway's content is a sign that the care pathway is being used as a reflective/best practice tool.

Benefits of variation reporting

- It is an in-built system for monitoring individual patient's/user's progress.
- It allows clinical staff to immediately identify if a patient/user is not following the anticipated or expected process.
- When aggregated, it allows clinical staff to methodically analyse the reasons for patient/user deviations when on the care pathway.
- It can be used to monitor performance.
- It can identify areas for service improvement.
- It promotes a 'continuous quality improvement' ethos.
- It minimises ad hoc 'one-off' audits on specific aspects of care.
- It identifies areas for future research.

These benefits can be linked to organisational goals of:

- clinical governance
- clinical audit
- clinical effectiveness
- implementation of evidence-based practice.

Uses of variation

There are two uses of variation reporting. These are:

- concurrent review
- retrospective review.

Concurrent review of variation

This is used by the staff delivering the care to individual patients/users as a day-to-day management tool. It provides a mechanism for the staff to see if the patient/user is progressing as expected. It highlights if this is not the case and allows the clinical staff to individualise the care pathway or to make a decision whether to take corrective action to get the patient/user back on the care pathway. Clinical and professional judgement must still be applied to decide what action to take for the individual patient/user.

Retrospective review of variation

The retrospective analysis of the variation for a number of patients/users is vital for 'closing the audit loop'. It enables staff to look at the results of the operation of the care pathway on a number of patients/users, and to identify trends. The multidisciplinary staff can then identify what action should be taken to improve care for a group of patients/users.

What to record as a variation

One of the fundamental principles advised is that *any variation from the care pathway for an individual patient/user must be recorded.* This information should include:

- details of the variation
- what action has been taken
- date/time
- signature of person completing variation information.

This information is essential to show how the care pathway has been adapted for individual patient/user circumstances or to show at which point the patient/user did not follow the expected or anticipated plan. This information is used primarily for the management and review of the *individual* patient/user.

In addition, you may wish to identify 'key events' or 'milestone/ indicators' and list these in the care pathway. These should be kept to a minimum (say, 10–15 maximum) but would reflect the development team's identification of what it feels are the essential clinical patient/user indicators it wishes to monitor and track. These key indicators usually comprise some form of clinical or process outcome wherever possible.

They should be monitored retrospectively and reviewed by the development group regularly.

An example of some key events/milestone indicators is shown in Box 4.1 for a chest pain and myocardial infarction care pathway.

Box 4.1: Key indicator/milestone for a chest pain myocardial infarction care pathway

- Time/date of onset of pain or other major symptoms.
- Time/date of call for help (either GP or ambulance).
- Time/date of arrival in A&E department.
- Time/date of commencement of thrombolytic therapy.
- Which thrombolytic agent did patient receive?
  Streptokinase/Reteplase/None
  If none please give brief details
- Did patient suffer any adverse effects from thrombolysis?
  If yes please give brief details
- Were intravenous beta-blockers given? *If no please give reason*
- Have beta blockers been prescribed as discharge medication?
  If no please give reason
- Has patient had an exercise test while in hospital?
  If not please give reason
- How many days has patient spent in hospital? *If longer than 6 days, please give reason.*

Source: Adapted from Worcestershire Acute Hospitals NHS Trust.

Now you identify some key indicators/outcomes/goals you want to monitor retrospectively in your care pathway.

Key indicator/milestone/goal

Coding of variations

Some organisations have found coding their variations useful when they come to retrospectively analyse them. A common coding categorisation refers to source of variation,[1] for example:

- *patient/user*: something the patient/user did or did not do
- *carer*: for example, unavailable to do the task specified
- *system*: some reason a task could not be done which is system-based, e.g. department closed, faulty equipment, equipment not available.

An alternative coding system might look at the categories of care.[1] For example:

- tests
- assessments

- consultations
- education
- discharge planning.

However, if a coding system is to be used, care needs to be taken to ensure the codes are applied consistently.

Consistent style to report variations

The decision on choice of method to record variation should take account of local circumstances. However, different variation reporting systems within one organisation are likely to become confusing when staff have to use multiple care pathways. A corporate or 'house style' is probably a necessity in this situation to avoid confusion. Consider asking your steering group to develop a template to record variations.

Presentation of variation analysis results

Various computer tools can be used to assist with the analysis of variation, e.g. Excel, Access. Some organisations also use scanning equipment to process their variations.

Consideration needs to be given to how the analysis should be presented. Graphs, 'run charts' and Pareto diagrams (the 80:20 rule) are effective presentation methods.

There is much written about the presentation of this type of data. If the reader wishes to read more on this subject a useful reference is:

- NHS Executive (1995) *Leading Improvement in Healthcare: a resource guide for process improvement.* DoH, London.

> **Box 4.2:** Useful tips
>
> - Ensure your care pathway documentation identifies who should record the variations.
> - Choose a mechanism to report variations – decide on a 'house style' to minimise confusion by staff when multiple care pathways are in use.
> - Coincide the reporting of variation analysis with staff changes. In the context of hospitals, this might be at junior doctor changeover. This helps to raise the profile that care pathways exist and shows that their audit is pivotal.

Reference

1 Potter P (1995) The uses of variance. K Zander (ed) *Managing Outcomes through Collaborative Care: the application of care mapping and case management.* American Hospital Publishing Inc., Illinois, pp 131–48.

Chapter 5

Implementation of a care pathway

Training of staff

The key to any pilot is *informing and training staff* who are going to use the care pathway of both the process changes in the delivery of care that will result from its use and any documentation changes.

Who does the training?

It is recommended that the individual members of the development group undertake the detailed training of staff who are about to use the care pathway.

These individuals are familiar with the care pathway and are best placed to explain the rationale and background to its contents.

What to cover when training staff to use the care pathway

The training will need to cover the following aspects of care pathway use:

- placing a patient/user on a care pathway and when to take them off
- examples of a well-completed pathway with variation-reporting mechanism
- examples of a poorly completed pathway and reasons why

- the need for signatures, where and what to write; what a signature implies
- no documentation – no defence
- reporting of variations
- use of the documentation for 'shift' handover purposes
- where the care pathway is to be stored
- how and when the variation reporting information will be analysed and reported.

Provide written instructions on how to use the care pathway and details of who to contact if they have problems.

Pilot (testing) the care pathway

Identify a start and end point of the pilot

Identify a start and end date for the pilot or specific number of patients/ users you want to go through on the care pathway before reviewing it (e.g. 10–15 patients/users). Make sure the pilot phase is not too long. Early feedback of the variations and use of the care pathway to the staff on how it is working is vital.

Facilitator and members of the development group to support the staff

Actively support the staff during the pilot. Visit the ward, GP practice, etc., regularly. Examine the care pathway documentation as it is being used. You will need to report the compliance in terms of completing the care pathway documentation at the pilot review meeting.

Count the number of patients/users who should have been put on the care pathway

Identify a method to count the number of patients/users with the particular condition/treatment who **should** be put on to the care pathway during the pilot, and compare this with the number of care pathway documents you review at the end of the pilot. By doing this you will know if staff are ignoring the care pathway and continuing with their old clinical documentation.

How to deal with issues/problems

Inevitably, there will be issues and problems to start with. If these are relatively minor in nature, then note them down ready to report to the development group at its review of the pilot. If major concerns arise, discuss them with members of the development group and decide whether to make changes to the care pathway or to halt the pilot. Changes to the care pathway documentation are common following a pilot of the tool.

Review of the pilot

At the review of the pilot, you will need information on:

- compliance with using the care pathway documentation
- information on the variations
- achievement of any standards or outcomes monitored as part of the care pathway
- a list of staff comments and problems with the care pathway.

Requests for changes in the care pathway at this point are a positive sign that staff are 'taking ownership' of the care pathway and testing the tool out.

Review check list

Table 5.1 is a check list of things to be considered when planning the pilot.

Table 5.1

Feature to check	Checked
• Start date of pilot	☐
• End date of pilot	☐
• Number of patients/users (throughput) of pilot (is it an adequate number?)	☐
• How is data for review to be collected?	
– compliance with care pathway documentation	☐
– variance reporting mechanism	☐
– standards/outcomes achieved	☐
– clinical staff opinions	☐
• Nominate person(s) responsible for collecting review data	☐
• Analysis of review data to be completed within . . . . weeks of end of pilot	☐
• Nominate person(s) responsible for analysing review data	☐
• Identify date for feedback of results of pilot to clinical staff	☐

Sign-off the care pathway

Within the context of clinical governance, it is important to ensure that your care pathway gains approval for use by the organisation(s) who will be using it. Many trusts ask for an individual care pathway to be appraised in terms of:

• content

• documentation design

• development process used.

Box 5.1: Useful tips

- Make sure old copies of the documentation are removed so that staff always use the latest version.
- Encourage senior staff to be seen to be actively supporting the early stages of the pilot.
- Put up an anonymous comment sheet for staff to write down any comments they may have about the care pathway.
- Don't delay the pilot in order to refine the documentation endlessly – there will always be changes as a result of the pilot.

Chapter 6

Maintaining the care pathway

On-going maintenance of the care pathway

From reading this resource guide, you will appreciate that, in a sense, no individual care pathway is ever finished, but remains a continually evolving tool.

Maintaining the continued use of a care pathway once developed and successfully implemented can be one of the hardest stages of all. Healthcare organisations have reported care pathways falling into disuse once the facilitator has moved on and refocused on a new care pathway condition.

If the care pathway is going to be maintained and used to promote a continuous improvement ethos, resources/individuals must be identified with specific responsibility for maintaining the care pathway. *Care pathways do not run on their own.*

Check list to maintain the momentum

Table 6.1 is a check list of what we believe are essential elements which need to be in place to ensure continued use of a care pathway.

Table 6.1

Features to be checked	Checked
• Nominate lead person for the maintenance of the care pathway	☐
• Robust arrangements in place for the production of the care pathway paper documentation or update procedure (if electronic)	☐
• Nominate person responsible for ensuring supplies of the documentation are available	☐
• On-going training programme in place for new staff	☐
• Person(s) nominated to provide training to new staff	☐
• An agreed audit plan and timetable in place including:	
– identification of what is to be audited	☐
– start and end dates of audit	☐
– number of patients/users (throughput)	☐
– person responsible for collecting data	☐
– person responsible for reporting data	☐
• Programme of multidisciplinary meetings to audit results is established	☐
• There is an agreed review date of care pathway content	☐

And finally . . . you know you have done a good job when . . .

- A consultant asks for a pathway to be developed on . . .
- The multidisciplinary team have gone and done more pathways than they were asked to do.
- If you had a vote, the staff would vote to continue to use care pathways rather than return to care planning.

Chapter 7

Troubleshooting guide

It is difficult to find specific pieces of information/sections in the care pathway document.
Consider dividing different sections of the care pathway document or colour-coding sections so those specific pieces can be found more easily.

Some care pathway sites have found it beneficial to introduce summary sheets at strategic stages of the care pathway (particularly at key interfaces, e.g. acute to community). This seems to work well if the condition covered by the care pathway is complex and covers a long period of time or covers a lot of departments/disciplines.

The documentation is large and cumbersome.
All members of the multidisciplinary group need to be vigilant to avoid this problem. They must continually question the necessity of including aspects of documentation. One of the key benefits of having multi-disciplinary documentation is that all staff have access. This should reduce the amount of information to be collected, as some of it only needs to be collected once.

Experience suggests that a certain 'trimming down' and shortening of the documentation is likely to occur after the pilot of the newly developed care pathway. This happens as staff begin to work with the documentation in a practical way and realise what information is of use to them and what is not.

Consider splitting the documentation into sections to be inserted as the patient/user progresses along the care pathway.

It looks like the documentation [insert particular professional group] use.
The danger that the documentation designed as part of the care pathway will look like the documentation for one particular discipline is something

the facilitator needs to be aware of. The documentation designed needs to be relevant to all disciplines involved.

The care pathway mapping process is getting very complicated with lots of possible routes patients/users may go down.
Think about splitting the care pathway into phases or stages. Alternatively, develop different care pathways for different sub-groups of patients/users.

Also, keep in mind that the care pathway is intended only for the majority of patients/users with a particular condition/disease. Remember the 80:20 rule. You are trying to develop a care pathway that will cover 80% of the patients/users in your group. A separate care pathway can cater for small subsets of patients/users within an overall condition/disease. For example, burns patients who go into toxic shock can have a separate care pathway for this particular situation.

A small group of individuals on the development group are dominating the discussions.
Be alert to the possibility of certain personalities dominating the process of development despite other disciplines' representation at developmental meetings. Make sure all disciplines contribute actively to the development meetings. The care pathway has to be relevant and meaningful to all disciplines involved. The need to keep some staff quiet while drawing others out is a vital skill of the facilitator.

Previous meetings may not have achieved much and been a free for all.
Ensure you are prepared – have an agenda with allocated timescales and stick to it. If two people cannot agree, discuss the item outside the meeting and get them to come back to you with the outcome. Provide timely minutes with action points and dates by which action is to be achieved.

Do you develop a care pathway that reflects current practice or 'best practice'?
There are two schools of thought. The first argues that it is better to develop a care pathway that reflects what can be achieved locally. In this way, the staff who are actually going to use it maintain ownership of the tool. The alternative view is that it is better to provide a 'gold standard', which the staff can work towards. The danger with this latter approach is

that staff get demotivated if they are given unrealistic targets and can quickly stop using them.

In practice, we have found that you usually end up with a combination of the two approaches. You need to examine each individual issue/problem and assess the benefits of reflecting current practice in this version of the care pathway (recognising that the care pathway will be regularly updated and changed anyway).